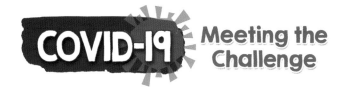

The COVID-19 Pandemic

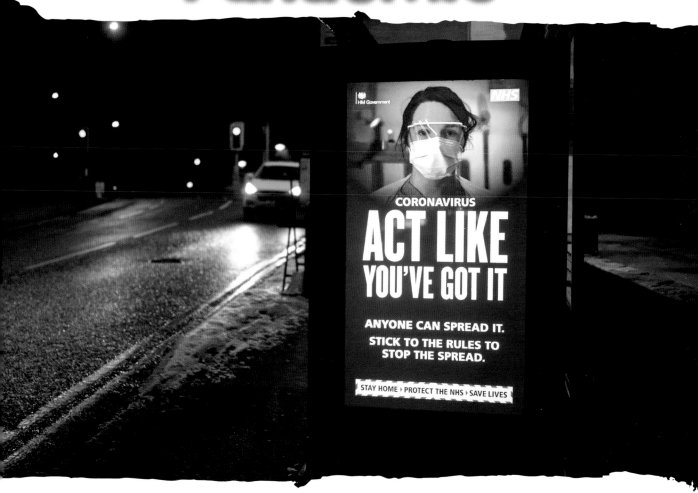

Samantha Kohn

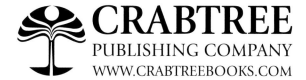

CRABTREE
PUBLISHING COMPANY
WWW.CRABTREEBOOKS.COM

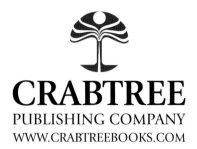

CRABTREE
PUBLISHING COMPANY
WWW.CRABTREEBOOKS.COM

Author:
Samantha Kohn

Series research and development:
Janine Deschenes and Ellen Rodger

Editorial director:
Kathy Middleton

Editor:
Janine Deschenes and Ellen Rodger

Proofreader:
Wendy Scavuzzo

Graphic design:
Samara Parent

Image research:
Samara Parent

Print coordinator:
Katherine Berti

Images:
Alamy
  coronavirus new york: p. 3
  REUTERS: p. 4 (bottom)
  Aflo Co. Ltd.: p. 4-5
  dpa picture alliance: p. 13 (bottom)
  ZUMA Press, Inc: p. 24
  Cavan Images: p. 26-27 (top)
  Science Photo Library: p. 33 (top)
  Tim Cordell: p. 35
  Ian Pilbeam: p. 38-39
  Cultura Creative Ltd: p. 40-41

Chris Leary Photography: p. 33 (bottom)

Shutterstock
  Jorge hely veiga: front cover (bottom)
  Matthew Troke: title page
  Thomas La Mela: p. 6-7
  Enrique Campo Bello: p. 9
  Alexandros Michailidis: p. 10 (bottom)
  Rob Hainer: p. 10-11

Steve Todd: p. 14
Javier Badosa: p. 15
BW Press: p. 16-17
Photocarioca: p. 17 (bottom)
kandl stock: p. 18 (bottom)
Tada Images: p. 18-19
Jillian Cain Photography: p. 20-21 (top)
Sebastian Reategui: p. 21 (bottom)
Wild Bite: p. 22 (bottom)
AlexiRosenfeld: p. 22-23
glen photo: p. 25
WoodysPhotos: p. 28-29 (top)
Paolo Bona: p. 28 (bottom)
LegoCamera: p. 30 (bottom)
bmszealand: p. 30-31 (top)
Rapture700: p. 31 (bottom)
Frederic Legrand - COMEO: p. 34
Blueee77: p. 39 (bottom)
Sundry Photography: p. 43 (top)
Joaquin Corbalan P: p. 45

All other images by Shutterstock

Library and Archives Canada Cataloguing in Publication

Title: The COVID-19 pandemic / Samantha Kohn.
Names: Kohn, Samantha, author.
Description: Series statement: COVID-19: meeting the challenge | Includes
  bibliographical references and index.
Identifiers: Canadiana (print) 20210214759 | Canadiana (ebook) 20210214767
| ISBN 9781427156020 (hardcover)
| ISBN 9781427156044 (softcover)
| ISBN 9781427156068 (HTML)
| ISBN 9781427156389 (EPUB)
Subjects: LCSH: COVID-19 Pandemic, 2020-—Juvenile literature. | LCSH:
  COVID-19 (Disease)—Juvenile
literature. | LCSH: COVID-19 Pandemic, 2020-—Social aspects—Juvenile
literature. | LCSH:
COVID-19 (Disease)—Social aspects—Juvenile literature.
Classification: LCC RA644.C67 K65 2022 | DDC j616.2/414—dc23

Library of Congress Cataloging-in-Publication Data

Names: Kohn, Samantha, author.
Title: The COVID-19 pandemic / Samantha Kohn.
Description: New York, NY : Crabtree Publishing Company, [2022] | Series:
  COVID-19: meeting the challenge | Includes index.
Identifiers: LCCN 2021020826 (print) | LCCN 2021020827 (ebook)
| ISBN 9781427156020 (hardcover)
| ISBN 9781427156044 (paperback)
| ISBN 9781427156068 (ebook)
| ISBN 9781427156389 (epub)
Subjects: LCSH: COVID-19 (Disease)--Juvenile literature. |
  Epidemics--Juvenile literature. | Diamond Princess
Classification: LCC RA644.C67 K642 2022 (print) | LCC RA644.C67 (ebook) |
  DDC 614.5/92414--dc23
LC record available at https://lccn.loc.gov/2021020826
LC ebook record available at https://lccn.loc.gov/2021020827

Crabtree Publishing Company

www.crabtreebooks.com 1-800-387-7650

Published in Canada
Crabtree Publishing
616 Welland Ave.
St. Catharines, Ontario
L2M 5V6

Published in the United States
Crabtree Publishing
347 Fifth Ave
Suite 1402-145
New York, NY 10016

Printed in the U.S.A./092021/CG20210616

CONTENTS

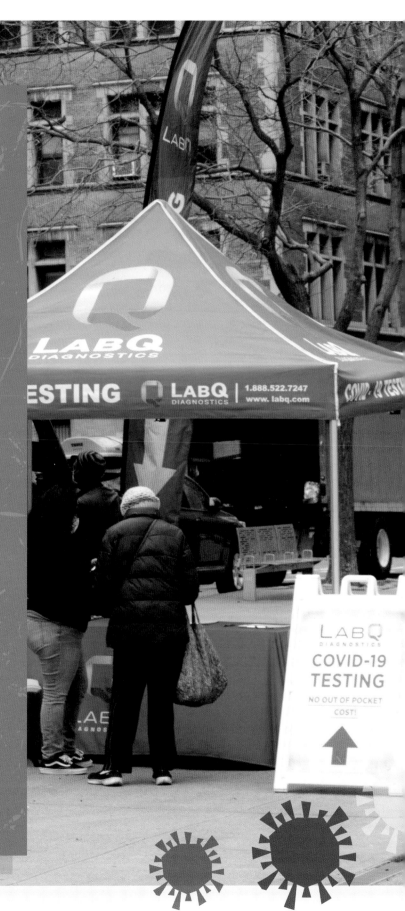

Introduction

When passengers and crew boarded the Diamond Princess cruise ship, they had no idea their luxury winter vacation would turn into a nightmare of **quarantine**, sickness, and death. The ship left Japan on January 20, 2020, for a 14-day round trip around Southeast Asia. Six days into the trip, one passenger tested positive with a new, unknown virus.

On the same day the Diamond Princess set sail, China's Center for Disease Control had shared news about a virus that was causing illness and death in the country. The new illness began in Wuhan, China in December, 2019. It was a **respiratory** disease that would later be named COVID-19. China classified the illness as a Class B **infectious** disease. That meant it could spread from person to person easily. January 20, 2020, was also the day that the first case of COVID-19 was reported in the United States.

On February 20, 2020, the Diamond Princess was docked at Yokahama, Japan. Its 3,711 passengers and crew had been confined to the ship for one month. Half of the world's known cases of COVID-19 were aboard. In total, more than 700 people on the cruise ship were infected with the virus and 14 died. The Diamond Princess was a lesson in COVID-19 safety. Epidemiologists, or the scientists who study diseases, learned that this new disease spread easily and quickly. It hit the elderly hard, but its spread could be controlled through strict quarantine.

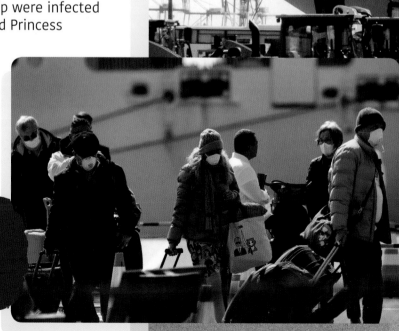

Passengers were allowed to disembark, or leave, the ship after they were tested for COVID-19 in early March 2020.

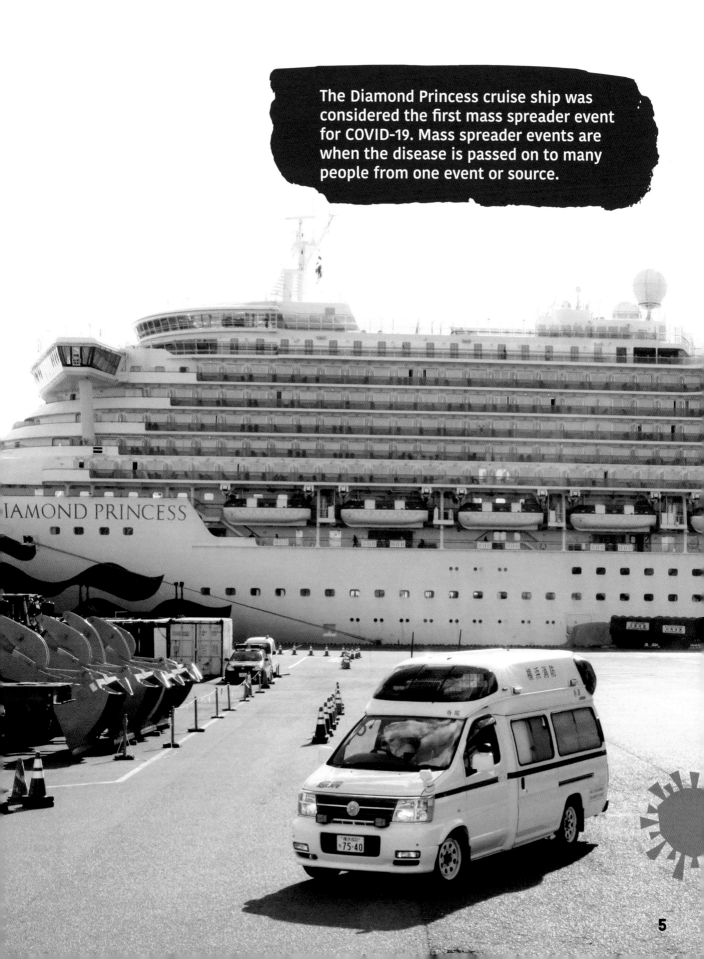

The Diamond Princess cruise ship was considered the first mass spreader event for COVID-19. Mass spreader events are when the disease is passed on to many people from one event or source.

A Virus Emerges

Coronaviruses are spread by **respiratory droplets**. These are **microscopic** splatters of saliva or mucous produced when humans exhale, talk, sneeze, or even sing. In other words, they are **airborne** droplets that cannot be seen by the naked eye.

Once a coronavirus makes its way inside a person, the spikes of the virus act like a key. They lock onto human **cells**. Coronaviruses are bossy—telling other cells to make copies. The virus copies itself over and over again inside the person unlucky enough to have breathed it in.

Easily Spread

The SARS-CoV-2 coronavirus that caused COVID-19 spread incredibly fast. Humans carried it throughout the world as they traveled. Because it was a novel, or new, virus, at first doctors and scientists knew little about how it spread. Over time, they learned how to best treat the people who were ill.

Respiratory droplets can land about 4–6 feet (1–2 m) away from a person. That could be on the ground, on a shelf at the store, or right onto another person nearby.

Coronaviruses got their name because of their spiky corona, or crown, seen under a microscope.

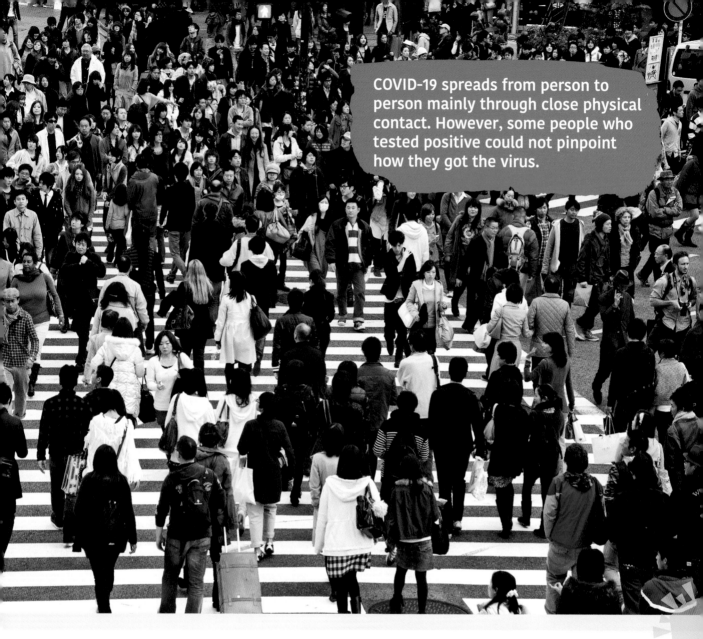

COVID-19 spreads from person to person mainly through close physical contact. However, some people who tested positive could not pinpoint how they got the virus.

Symptoms and Spread

Two things about COVID-19 make it hard to control. First, people with COVID-19 are **contagious** before they start feeling **symptoms**. This means that many people spread the virus before knowing that they have it. Each infected person infects an average of two to three other people, who then go on to infect two to three others, and so on. That causes what's called **exponential spread**. The second problem is that most COVID-19 symptoms are fairly common. At first, many people found it difficult to tell whether their headaches and sore throats meant they should get tested for COVID-19.

At the beginning of the **pandemic**, people were told to assess themselves for symptoms of COVID-19 before leaving the house. These symptoms included a cough, fever, and shortness of breath. Within a few months, the list of symptoms had grown to include fatigue, aches and pains, sore throat, diarrhea, ringing ears, and the loss of taste or smell. Even more symptoms were added over time. Some of them were odd, such as a mental cloudiness called brain fog. Symptoms in children included rashes and "COVID toes," or toes that were red and purple colored.

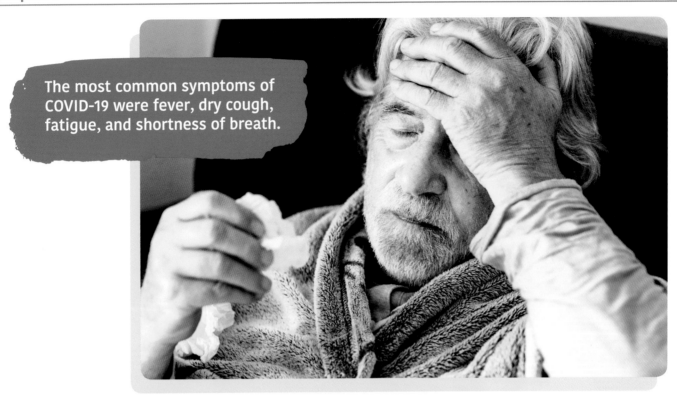

The most common symptoms of COVID-19 were fever, dry cough, fatigue, and shortness of breath.

Who's at Risk?

It was impossible to know who would get the virus and who would get really sick from it. One person could get it and feel okay, or just a bit unwell. But another could get it and spend weeks in the hospital. Some died. People from every age group, fitness level, and race have become seriously ill and died from COVID-19. Although anyone can become ill from COVID-19, scientists soon discovered that there were two groups who were at greater risk of serious COVID-19. Those were the elderly and people with **chronic** or serious illnesses such as diabetes or kidney disease.

The Most Vulnerable

In the **first wave** of COVID-19, in late 2020 to early 2021, the virus proved more deadly for people over the age of 65. Eight out of ten COVID-19 deaths in the United States were in people from that age group. According to the **World Health Organization (WHO)**, this is because of changes that happen as people get older or develop health conditions. In Canada, long-term care homes for the elderly had 69 percent of the country's COVID-19 deaths— mostly in the first wave.

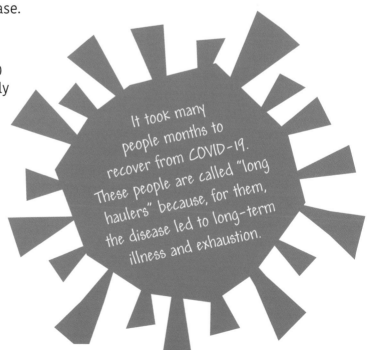

It took many people months to recover from COVID-19. These people are called "long haulers" because, for them, the disease led to long-term illness and exhaustion.

Health Conditions

During the first months of the pandemic, it was common to hear the term "underlying health conditions" used to describe those with increased risk. This referred to health problems a person had before they caught COVID-19. One study showed COVID-19 patients with underlying medical conditions, such as heart disease and diabetes, were hospitalized six times as often as people without. They were also 12 times more likely to die. As the pandemic lengthened, more contagious COVID-19 **variants** emerged. Those variants infected many younger and healthier people, including pregnant women.

PANDEMIC WHO'S WHO

Maria Branyas

Maria Branyas was a 113-year old woman living in a long-term care home near Barcelona, Spain. When she became infected with COVID-19, she was thought to be the oldest woman in Spain. Branyas got sick during Spain's first major outbreak in March 2020. At that point in her long life, Branyas had been through a lot. Even though her age put her at high risk of dying from COVID-19, she fought the illness and survived. This was one more triumph added to her amazing life story. Branyas was born in 1907, which meant she also lived through two world wars and the 1918–1919 flu pandemic, also known as the Spanish flu. That pandemic killed 50 million people worldwide. After becoming infected with COVID-19, Branyas spent weeks quarantined in her room with mild symptoms.

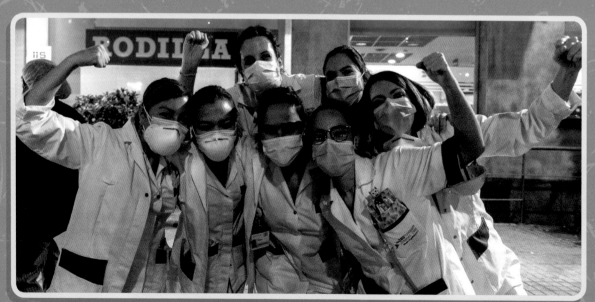

Spanish health care workers pose for a group photo during COVID-19.

Who's in Charge

The world was shocked by the fast-moving COVID-19 pandemic. But there have been pandemics before—five in the last 100 years! COVID-19 was the first in many decades to spread so widely and so quickly. Governments around the world rolled out plans to deal with the virus. Plans included imposing **lockdowns**, and making sure countries had enough personal protective equipment (PPE), such as masks and gloves. While governments around the world rolled out their own plans to deal with COVID-19, there were two main organizations that the world looked to for information about this pandemic.

WHO to Turn To

The WHO is a special agency of the United Nations. It is responsible for **public health** around the world. It has a headquarters in Geneva, Switzerland, and regional offices around the world. The WHO monitors public health risks such as emerging viruses and diseases. It also coordinates responses to these health emergencies. The WHO has 194 member countries and their funding keeps the organization running.

Throughout the pandemic, the WHO put together information on how COVID-19 was affecting countries all over the world.

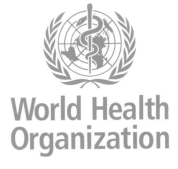

World Health Organization

During COVID-19, governments and people around the world looked to the WHO and its leader Tedros Adhanom Ghebreyesus for information about the pandemic. This included how and where it was spreading, and updates on vaccines.

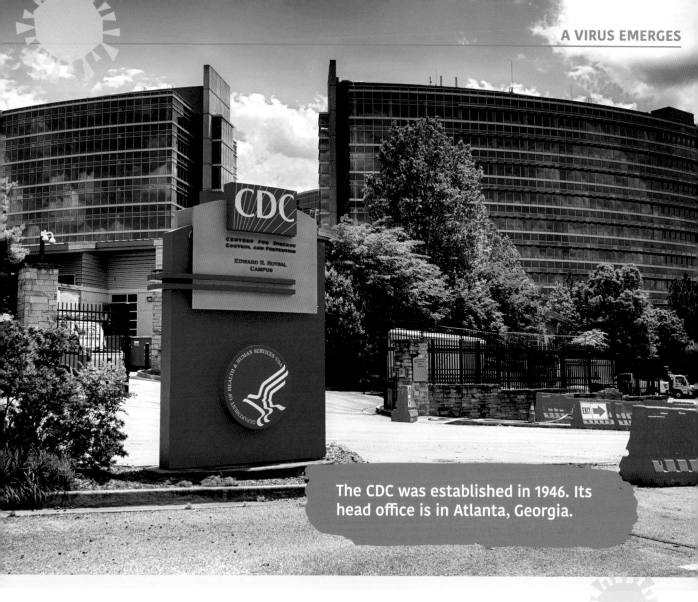

The CDC was established in 1946. Its head office is in Atlanta, Georgia.

Centers for Disease Control and Prevention

The Centers for Disease Control and Prevention, or the CDC, is part of the United States Department of Health & Human Services. Their mission is to protect America from health, safety, and security threats. Some of those threats, such as pandemics, are international. The CDC works with state and local health departments to discover disease patterns. That includes where diseases are spreading, who they're spreading to, and the impact that those diseases have.

Information Sharing

A major part of the CDC's job is sharing information. During the COVID-19 pandemic, people looked to the CDC for information on the virus and how it was spreading. As scientists learned more, such as what treatments were effective, the CDC published that information. That ensured people had the most up-to-date recommendations based on known science.

A Spreading Virus

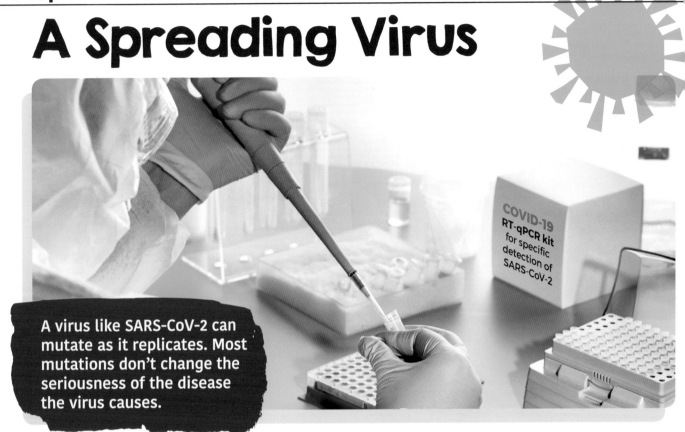

A virus like SARS-CoV-2 can mutate as it replicates. Most mutations don't change the seriousness of the disease the virus causes.

Many viruses don't make their **hosts** very sick. People infected with those viruses feel normal, so they carry on with their day-to-day lives. That means they can spread the virus without even knowing it.

Viruses cannot live and **reproduce** on their own. They need a host to live in or on. Viruses are not considered living things because they have no **cells**. They survive by replicating or copying in the cells of hosts. If a virus runs out of hosts, it dies. So viruses continually adapt to provide themselves with as many hosts as possible. These adaptations are called mutations. A virus with one or more mutations is called a variant.

Sometimes variants appear, then disappear. In just over a year, the SARS-CoV-2 virus that causes COVID-19 is estimated to have created many thousands of variants. Only a few are called "variants of concern." These are variants that have **evolved** to spread more easily or cause more severe symptoms. The biggest worry is that a vaccine created for the original virus is not effective against the variant.

Scientists believe that the virus that caused the COVID-19 pandemic was present in animals for some time. They think something happened in 2019 that caused the virus to mutate, or change. It began to latch onto human beings as its host, rather than animals.

A Novel Virus

The coronavirus that causes COVID-19 is new to humans. Doctors and scientists had never seen it before. At first, they were not sure what treatments, medicines, and **protocols** would work the best. So, they tried many different ideas.

Coronaviruses

Although COVID-19 was a new virus, it fell under a broader group of coronaviruses that cause disease in mammals and birds. There are seven coronaviruses known to affect humans. Some of those viruses cause illnesses that most people have recovered from many times in their lives. About 15 to 30 percent of cold viruses are coronaviruses, for example. Other coronaviruses cause more serious illnesses. Those include Severe Acute Respiratory Syndrome (SARS) and Middle East Respiratory Syndrome (MERS).

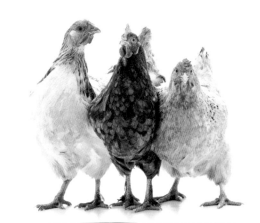

Research on coronaviruses has been going on since the 1930s, when scientists investigated a respiratory infection that killed chickens. Human coronaviruses were discovered in the 1960s.

PANDEMIC WHO'S WHO

Dr. Anthony Fauci

One of the most recognized faces and voices of the COVID-19 pandemic was Dr. Anthony Fauci. The American doctor and researcher specializes in the study of infectious diseases. Dr. Fauci is also the director of the U.S. National Institute of Allergy and Infectious Diseases. During COVID-19, Dr. Fauci was a member of the White House Coronavirus Task Force under President Donald Trump in 2020. He continued as a chief Medical Advisor to President Joseph Biden in 2021. Early in the pandemic, Dr. Fauci was described as one of the most trusted figures in the medical field. His advice reassured people at a time when the U.S. saw 2,000 to 3,000 COVID-19 deaths a day.

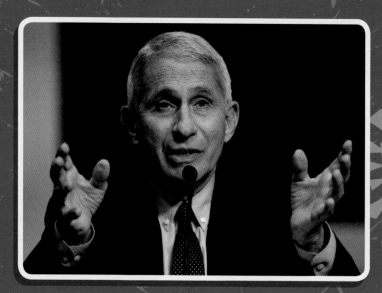

Dr. Fauci was an advisor to seven American presidents on national and global health issues.

Spreading Without Symptoms

People who were sick with COVID-19 were spreading the disease far and wide. Even those who stayed home had a good chance of spreading the disease to the people they lived with. If someone became sick enough to need medical care, nurses, doctors, and hospital staff were at risk of catching the virus from them.

Visibly sick COVID-19 patients weren't the only ones spreading the disease. People who were pre-symptomatic and asymptomatic could also spread the virus. That was one of the major reasons that COVID-19 became a global pandemic. Asymptomatic refers to people who are infected, but never develop any symptoms. Pre-symptomatic refers to infected people who have not developed symptoms yet, but will develop them later on. Much of the disease spread came from pre-symptomatic and asymptomatic people. Since those people often do not know they are infected, they go out in the world as normal. The virus is then exposed to more and more hosts.

New Zealand closed its borders to all but citizens, residents, and those with existing **visas**. It kept them closed for more than a year. People returning to the country had to quarantine in a hotel for two weeks at their own expense. The strict border closure helped control the spread of COVID-19 in that country.

New Zealand turned a military training base into a quarantine facility for New Zealanders returning from Wuhan, China in February 2020. They were placed in isolation for 14 days.

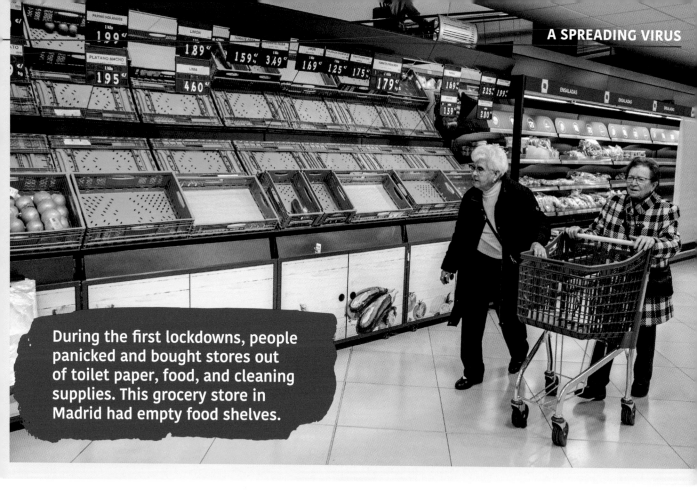

During the first lockdowns, people panicked and bought stores out of toilet paper, food, and cleaning supplies. This grocery store in Madrid had empty food shelves.

COVID-19 Research

Researchers and scientists published many studies about how likely it was for a COVID-19 carrier to spread the disease without feeling any symptoms. As new research came out, some of the things previously believed about the virus changed. That was one of the many issues in dealing with a new virus. At first, information was based on previous research and experience of how viruses and pandemics worked.

Lockdowns

Controlling the spread from asymptomatic people was one of the reasons that governments began lockdowns. Lockdowns aimed to control the spread by limiting contact between people. Borders were closed, and businesses and schools were closed or restricted. It wasn't enough to keep sick people at home, because sick people were not the only ones spreading the disease. Governments had to assume everyone could be a carrier of the virus. Keeping people apart was one important way to control the spread of the virus.

As scientists did more research on COVID-19, their findings helped public health officials give better advice to people. For example, public health advised the public to wear masks when it was determined that virus particles spread less easily when everyone wore masks.

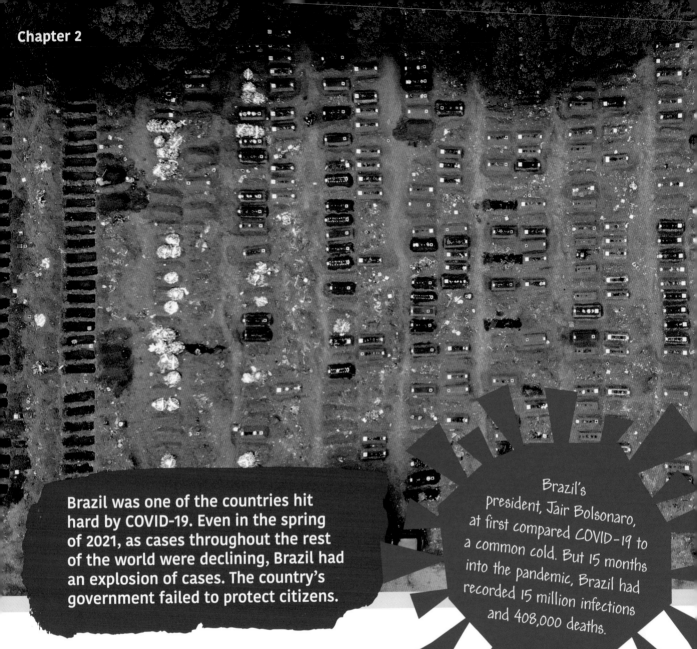

Brazil was one of the countries hit hard by COVID-19. Even in the spring of 2021, as cases throughout the rest of the world were declining, Brazil had an explosion of cases. The country's government failed to protect citizens.

Brazil's president, Jair Bolsonaro, at first compared COVID-19 to a common cold. But 15 months into the pandemic, Brazil had recorded 15 million infections and 408,000 deaths.

A Successful Virus

Common colds are one of the most successful viruses. Everybody has caught a cold at one time. Luckily, most colds don't make people very sick. Most people recover from colds within a week to 10 days. A few people could develop more serious symptoms, such as lung infections, but that is very unusual.

Easily Spread

Colds spread in much the same way as the virus that causes COVID-19. People sneeze, cough, and touch things. This sends the virus off into the world to find another host. Colds have been around for a long time. This makes them predictable. As a new-to-humans disease, COVID-19 was not predictable. While many people got seriously ill and some died from COVID-19, others only experienced mild symptoms. Some never felt any symptoms at all.

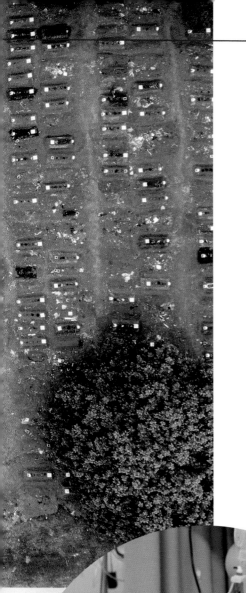

Epidemics and Pandemics

Other coronaviruses have caused serious illnesses and death over the past 20 years. Scientists warn that with **global warming**, **deforestation**, and increasing populations, the world will see more epidemics or pandemics of zoonotic origin. Zoonotic describes a disease that started in animals and "jumped" to the human population.

MERS

Like the COVID-19 virus, Middle East Respiratory Syndrome (MERS) was new to humans. Scientists believe it originated in animals, then evolved to spread to humans. MERS was first reported in Saudi Arabia in 2012. According to scientists, it may have started with bats, then was transmitted to camels and humans. It ultimately caused 858 deaths in 27 countries. The WHO believes 35 percent of people who contracted MERS died from the disease.

SARS

In 2003, another zoonotic disease emerged in China. The disease was called Severe Acute Respiratory Syndrome, better known as SARS. It eventually spread to more than two dozen countries before it was contained, or under control. SARS infected 8,098 people and killed 774 of them. It is believed that 14 to 15 percent of people infected with SARS did not survive. This made SARS less deadly than MERS. However, it spread farther because it was easier to spread.

> The full effects COVID-19 has on people's health is not yet known. Many people were still weak many months after surviving the disease. It may be that they have COVID-19-related health problems for the rest of their lives.

How COVID-19 Spread

COVID-19 started with one case in China. In less than a year, it had infected more than 100 million people. It caused more than 2 million deaths in nearly 200 countries in 2020 alone. And that was before mutations of the virus made it easier for the disease to infect people. The countries with the highest number of confirmed cases were the United States, India, and Brazil. These three countries were slow to recognize COVID-19 as a threat. That allowed the virus to spread widely until vaccine programs lessened its impact. Once COVID-19 vaccines were developed, the United States made up for lost time with the biggest vaccination campaign in world history. It averaged 21.1 million vaccinations per day by May 2021.

In the Beginning

March 11, 2020, was a day to remember. It was when the WHO announced that COVID-19 was a global pandemic. At that point, there were more than 118,000 cases in more than 110 countries around the world. It was clear that things would not be getting better any time soon.

At the beginning of the pandemic, disease experts said they expected COVID-19 to last 18 months to 2 years. The recovery from the pandemic will take longer.

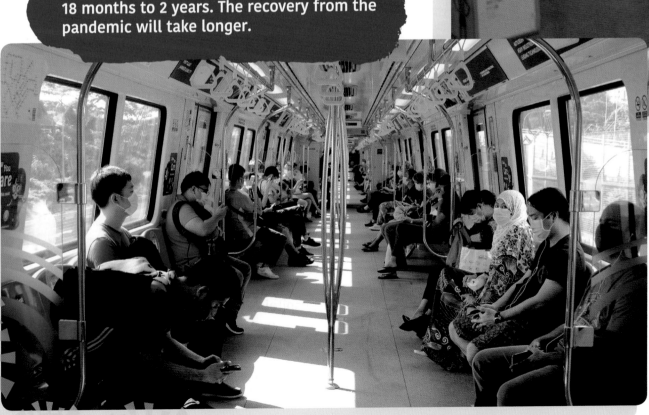

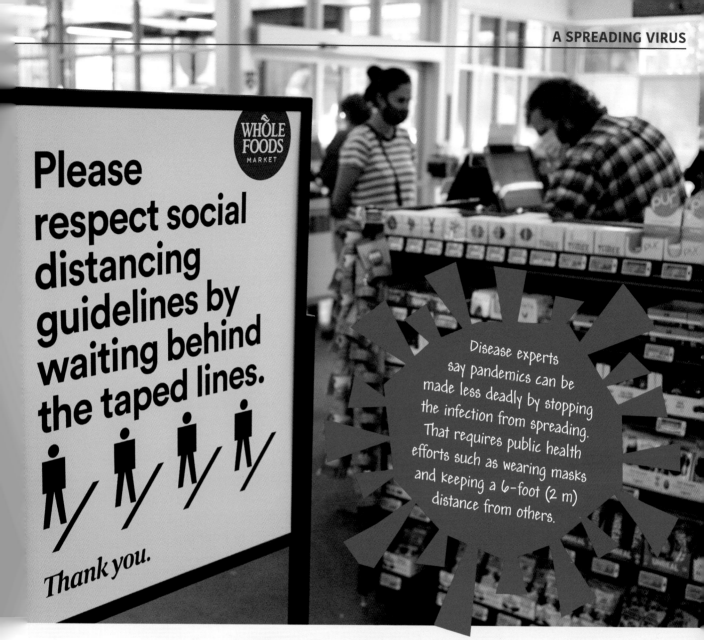

Please respect social distancing guidelines by waiting behind the taped lines.

Thank you.

WHOLE FOODS MARKET

Disease experts say pandemics can be made less deadly by stopping the infection from spreading. That requires public health efforts such as wearing masks and keeping a 6-foot (2 m) distance from others.

ow Did It Get Here?

uses don't travel great distances on their
n. But people do. The main reason that the
s that caused COVID-19 traveled around
world so quickly is that human beings often
vel internationally. In early 2020, it was just
easy for many people to get on a plane and
vel to another country as it was to get on a
and travel to a nearby city. In 1990, 1 billion
ple traveled by air. In 2018, that number was
rly 4 billion. With so many people traveling
oss the world every day, the new coronavirus
ead quickly.

Containment

Once the disease had spread to multiple
countries, keeping it contained was difficult.
Areas with high population densities, or where
many people live in a small amount of space,
saw higher spikes in cases. Big cities such as
New York City were some of the first to have
hospitals overwhelmed with the number of sick
patients. City dwellers were more likely to live
in apartment buildings and condominiums. They
also used public transportation. This meant
sharing elevators, subway cars, buses, cabs, and
other common spaces with many people.

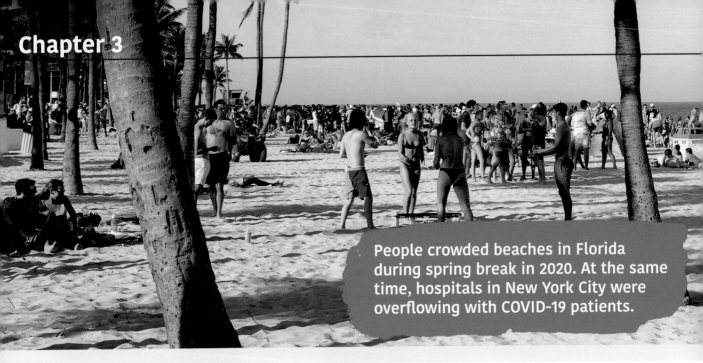

People crowded beaches in Florida during spring break in 2020. At the same time, hospitals in New York City were overflowing with COVID-19 patients.

The Global Response

The COVID-19 pandemic hit almost every corner of the world. Even places where there were no recorded cases were affected because we live in an interconnected world. Every government wanted to protect its people and its economy from the devastating impact of this virus, but they all had different plans on how to do that.

Imposing lockdowns was a main action governments took to slow the spread of COVID-19. A lockdown meant that people living in an area had to follow a set of rules aimed at keeping people away from one another. These rules included ordering people to stay at home. Usually, people were only allowed to leave for essential purposes, such as buying food. It also meant closing businesses such as restaurants, gyms, hair and nail salons, and more. By the first week of April 2020, more than half of the world's population was in some form of lockdown. Many people were working from computers at home. But not every job could be done at home. Many people were needed to work in grocery stores, food service industries, factories, hospitals, and home care. These people had to risk exposing themselves to the virus while traveling to and from work. They were also at risk at work.

Total Lockdowns

Total lockdowns meant that an entire country was placed under a new set of laws to encourage people to stay home and away from others. In some places, there were **curfews** to make sure people were in their homes by a certain time in the evening. These were used to prevent people from gathering together. Schools were closed to keep children apart from one another. Many international borders were closed, meaning people could not travel from one country to another.

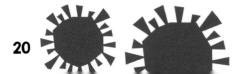

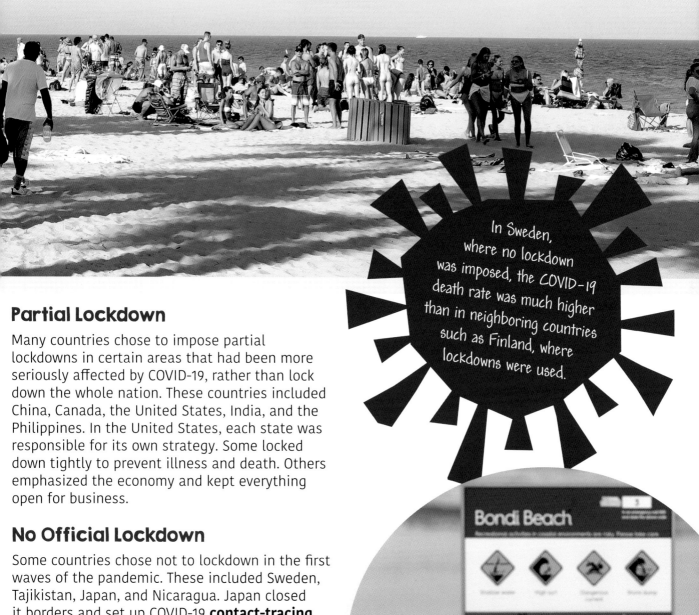

Partial Lockdown

Many countries chose to impose partial lockdowns in certain areas that had been more seriously affected by COVID-19, rather than lock down the whole nation. These countries included China, Canada, the United States, India, and the Philippines. In the United States, each state was responsible for its own strategy. Some locked down tightly to prevent illness and death. Others emphasized the economy and kept everything open for business.

No Official Lockdown

Some countries chose not to lockdown in the first waves of the pandemic. These included Sweden, Tajikistan, Japan, and Nicaragua. Japan closed it borders and set up COVID-19 **contact-tracing** programs. In early 2021, it declared a **state of emergency** in Tokyo after a surge in cases. The Central Asian country of Tajikistan declared itself COVID-19-free in January 2021. That declaration was believed to not be truthful.

In Sweden, where no lockdown was imposed, the COVID-19 death rate was much higher than in neighboring countries such as Finland, where lockdowns were used.

Each country had a different way of locking down their populations. Australia had few cases of COVID-19 in April 2020. However, its government still chose to set strict lockdown measures, including closing beaches such as Bondi Beach in Sydney, to prevent spread.

Italy

On March 2, 2020, the government of Italy declared a national lockdown. The country had record numbers of COVID-19 illnesses and hospitals were overflowing with the sick and dying. To try to limit the spread and save lives, Italy's government needed to keep people home. People were told not to leave their homes unless it was absolutely necessary. Necessary outings were for work, buying food, or health emergencies. All businesses were closed, except grocery stores and pharmacies. Even going out for a run was not allowed. Police patrolled the streets, sending people home who were out for **non-essential** reasons. That lockdown was especially difficult in a country where extended families often gathered for shared meals and celebrations.

New Zealand

New Zealand's first identified COVID-19 case was announced on February 28, 2020. By March 14, 2020, every person coming into the country had to go into self-isolation when they arrived. That meant they had to stay away from other people, even their families. A few days later, the borders were completely closed to non-citizens. By March 25, everyone living in New Zealand was put under a strict lockdown. People were asked to stay home. Non-essential businesses were closed. All workers who could work from home did so. By early June 2020, New Zealand had zero cases of COVID-19. Lockdown measures were lifted. Other than some **social distancing** recommendations, life went back to normal. When new cases popped up—from people traveling home from abroad—New Zealand's fast "test, trace, and isolate" plan kept these cases from spreading across the country.

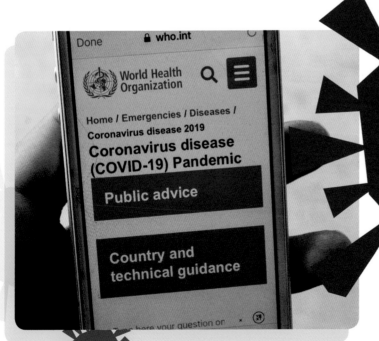

New Zealand used an alert system that listed four stages, or levels, of COVID-19 risk. Different lockdown measures applied to each stage. The country's overall COVID-19 plan also included a tracer app for cell phones. It helped people keep track of where they went, for contact tracing.

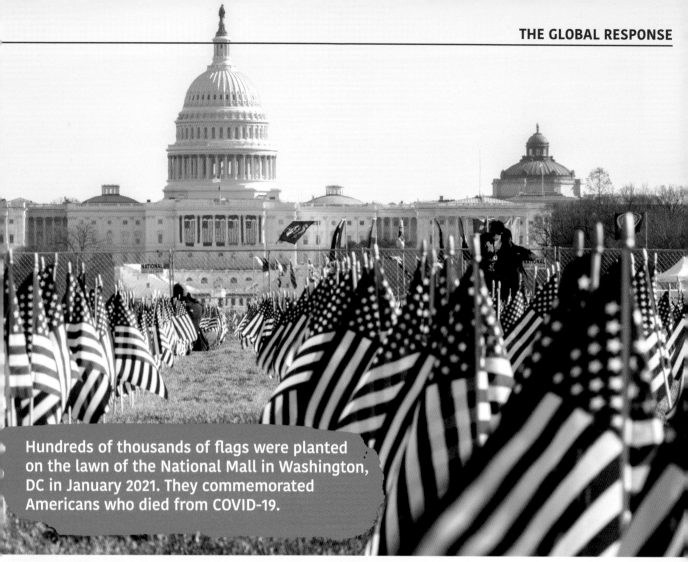

Hundreds of thousands of flags were planted on the lawn of the National Mall in Washington, DC in January 2021. They commemorated Americans who died from COVID-19.

The United States

The United States declared COVID-19 a public health emergency on February 3, 2020—weeks before the WHO announced it as a pandemic on March 11. By that time, the virus was already spreading. Travel bans were issued for non-U.S. citizens traveling from China and Europe. Lockdowns, however, were the responsibility of state governments. California was the first state to issue a stay-at-home order on March 19, 2020. Every state issued some COVID-19 protections, though 10 did not impose lockdowns. During March and April 2020, more than 310 million Americans were under some sort of COVID-19 rules. By May 2021, nearly 33 million people in the U.S. had become infected with COVID-19, and 577,046 had died.

Sweden

While most of the world stayed home during the first wave of COVID-19, life in Sweden stayed close to normal. While there was a temporary ban on gatherings of more than 50 people, and the government did recommend voluntary social distancing, Sweden did not shut down elementary schools, gyms, or restaurants. In fact, the government actively discouraged people from wearing masks. By spring 2021, Sweden's infection rates and deaths from COVID-19 were higher than any of their neighboring countries. Eventually, it became clear to government decision makers that letting the people of Sweden make their own decisions around how they would handle the pandemic was not working.

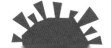

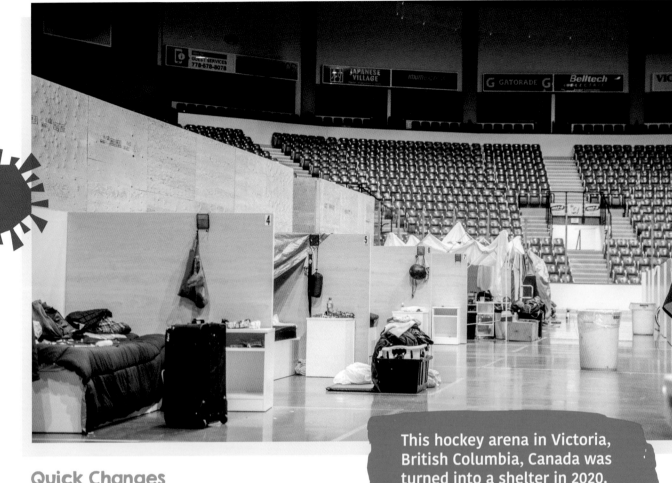

This hockey arena in Victoria, British Columbia, Canada was turned into a shelter in 2020. The shelter was one attempt to keep **unhoused** people safe during COVID-19.

Quick Changes

While the length and severity of the lockdowns were different depending where a person lived, most people in the world faced some sort of COVID-19 restrictions. In the early first wave, governments were not quite sure how to best protect citizens. By March 24, 2020, about 20 percent of the global population was living under lockdown. Within a week, it was half the world's population, or about 3.9 billion people.

Day-to-Day Life

Day-to-day life changed very quickly for so many people on lockdown. One day, they were setting their alarms to wake up for work or school. The next day, they rolled out of bed a few minutes before their first morning meeting or class. Work or school was now online, wherever possible. For some people, lockdowns simply meant a slower pace of life. However, the restrictions on daily life also created serious problems.

Out of Work

When non-essential businesses closed, that meant people working at hotels, airports, airlines, restaurants, hair salons, clothing stores, and cruise ships suddenly had no work to go to. In January 2020, about 3.6 percent of Americans were unemployed. By April, that number jumped to 14.7 percent. During lockdown measures, women had a higher rate of unemployment than men. That is because personal service jobs, held mostly by women, were shut down. Later, as global trade was interrupted, men's unemployment also rose.

Addictions

COVID-19 lockdowns and stay-at-home orders were especially difficult for people with addictions to drugs and alcohol. They were stuck at home or on the street, unable to access support such as therapy. Stress about the pandemic also affected their addictions. Experts described the increase in addiction and drug overdoses as another pandemic. In Ontario, Canada, **opioid** overdose deaths increased by 75 percent between December 2019 and March 2020, compared to the same time period the previous year. By August 2020, overdoses on opioids in large American cities had risen by 54 percent.

Violence in the Home

Before the pandemic, women and children had some distance from abusive partners and parents. They could leave home for work, school, or social outings. When lockdowns were imposed, that stopped. They were stuck at home with their abusers, and those abusers were more stressed than ever. This led to an increase in violence in the home. In early lockdown, intimate partner, or domestic violence reports increased by 30 percent in France, 25 percent in Argentina, and 18 percent in Spain. Things were similar in North America. For example, in Portland, Oregon, arrests related to domestic abuse rose by 22 percent.

PANDEMIC WHO'S WHO

Tsai Ing-Wen

Tsai Ing-Wen is the president of Taiwan, an island country 100 miles (160 km) off the coast of China. She was made one of *TIME* magazine's 100 most influential people of 2020, partly for her government's ability to keep the COVID-19 virus under control. As soon as COVID-19 reared its head in China, Tsai's administration took action to keep the country safe. Taiwan used its Central Epidemic Command Center (CECC) to coordinate its response. The CECC sent out text warnings to cell phones in the country. It controlled the distribution of PPE such as masks, and helped trace positive cases. The CECC was set up after the 2003–2004 SARS pandemic caused 181 deaths in Taiwan. Taiwan realized it needed a system that could keep its citizens from getting ill with the next pandemic. With COVID-19, Tsai Ing-Wen shut down Taiwan's borders and encouraged measures to prevent the disease from spreading. Her government set fines of up to $35,000 U.S. for people breaking COVID-19 rules. By the end of 2020, thecountry of 23 million people had just over 600 cases of COVID-19 and only 7 deaths.

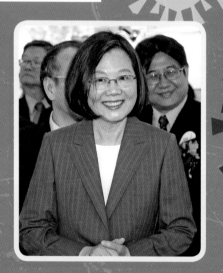

Tsai Ing-Wen helped create one of the world's most effective responses to COVID-19. Taiwan saw a rapid increase in cases only when the country started relaxing its restrictions in 2021, resulting in a national lockdown.

Flatten the Curve

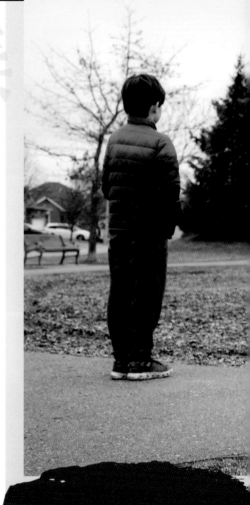

In the first few months of 2020, you couldn't watch a single news report or read an article about COVID-19 without hearing the words "flatten the curve." Flatten the curve means slowing down the spread of a disease so the health care system is not overwhelmed.

Many countries managed to flatten their curves in the first wave of COVID-19. However, numbers of COVID-19 cases increased steadily in countries such as the United States, Italy, the United Kingdom, and Brazil. In some areas, health care systems couldn't handle the number of people who needed hospitalization. Flattening the curve describes how slowing the spread of the virus, through measures such as hand washing, mask wearing, and social distancing, helps hospitals. A high curve means too many sick people in hospital at one time. A flatter curve means lower numbers of sick people, or that not everyone gets sick at the same time. The lower numbers take pressure off the hospitals.

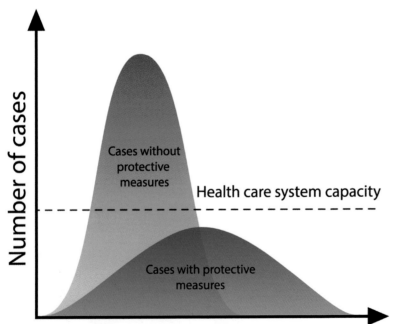

Cases without protective measures

Health care system capacity

Cases with protective measures

Number of cases

Time since first case

When too many people get seriously ill at once, health care systems cannot provide hospital care for everyone. The broken line shows the health care system capacity. This is the ability of hospitals to care for sick people. The red curve is an estimate of how many people would need care without lockdown restrictions. The blue curve is the estimate of how many people would need care if lockdown restrictions were imposed and followed.

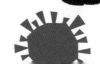

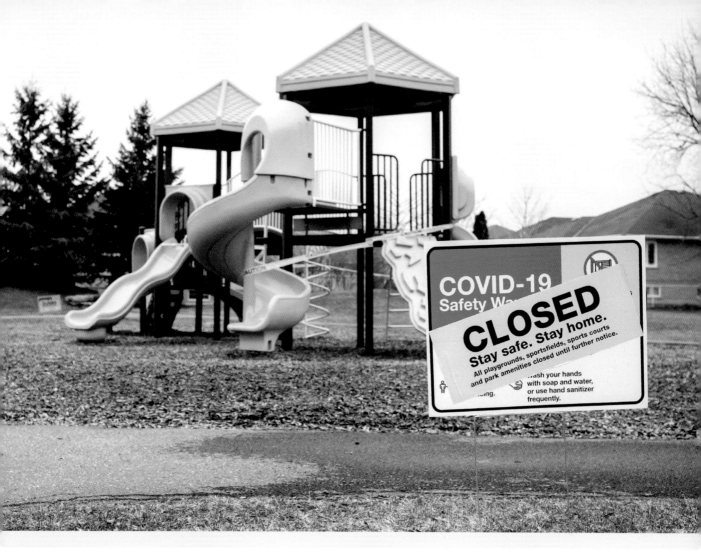

Public Health Measures

Public health is an area of health care that uses science to protect and improve the health of communities. These communities can be as small as one town, or as large as an entire country or region of the world. Government public health departments study and make recommendations on diseases and other things that affect health.

During the COVID-19 pandemic, public health had an important role in providing people with the latest information to protect them from getting the virus. Public health officials asked people to take precautions, such as washing their hands, staying home, wearing masks, and social distancing from other people. These simple things made it harder for the virus to transmit. Though experts knew people would get sick despite these measures, the hope was that taking precautions would mean fewer people getting sick all at once. That would help hospitals cope and allow for better treatment.

Scientists believed that 6 feet (2 m) was the distance that the virus droplets could travel when a person spoke, sang, coughed, or sneezed.

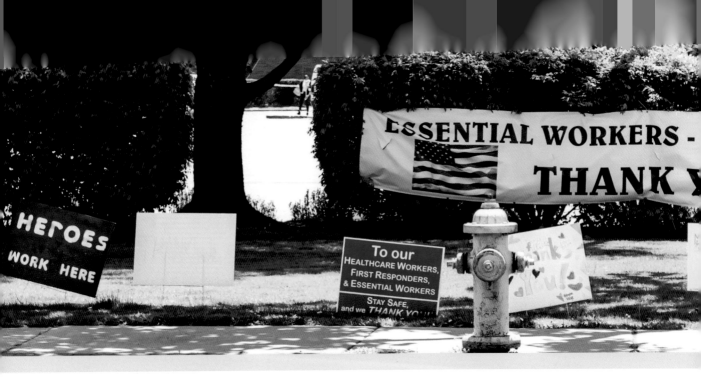

Challenged Health Care Systems

As more people became ill with COVID-19, health care systems around the world faced different levels of pressure. In January 2020, Chinese health officials knew that their hospitals would not be able to handle the number of COVID-19 patients needing care. Patients were being turned away because there weren't enough beds or supplies available. The Chinese government sprang into action faster than the world had ever seen. In just over one week, two new hospitals were built in the city of Wuhan—one with 1,000 beds and one with 1,600 beds.

New York's First Wave

In late March 2020, New York governor Andrew Cuomo shared that there were only 53,000 hospital beds available in the state. That was less than half of the 110,000 hospital beds the state predicted it would need to treat COVID-19 patients. That was a perfect example of the curve not being flattened to a level where the hospitals could care for all the patients in need. Hospitals across the state were ordered to increase their capacity. Non-essential surgeries were canceled, and New York City operating rooms were converted into intensive care units.

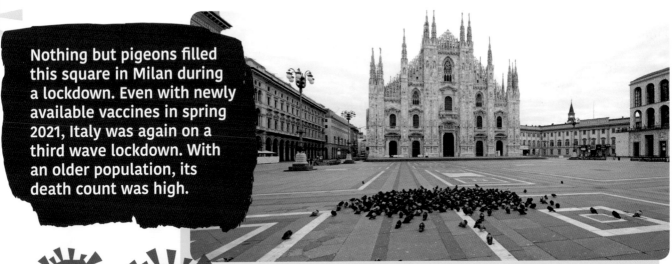

Nothing but pigeons filled this square in Milan during a lockdown. Even with newly available vaccines in spring 2021, Italy was again on a third wave lockdown. With an older population, its death count was high.

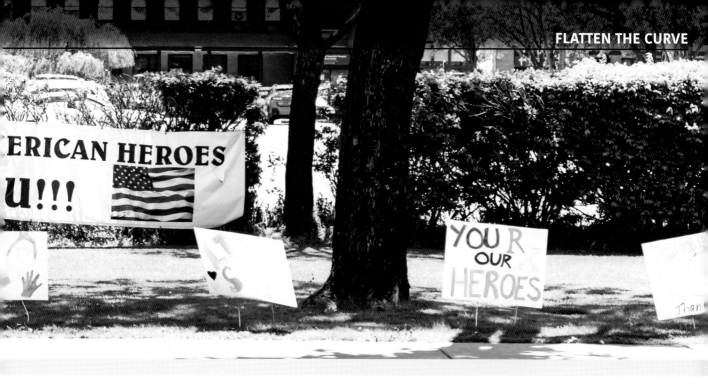

India's Second Wave

India's first confirmed COVID-19 case was in January 2020. The country of 1.4 billion people used a series of lockdowns in areas where the disease was spreading to try to keep it under control. In October 2020, a government panel said COVID-19 infections had peaked. A vaccination program began in January 2021. Then, new virus variants began to spread. The government had not prepared for that. It had even removed some temporary COVID-19 hospitals. By April 2021, things were out of control. Indian hospitals were overflowing. Supplies of oxygen ran out, and infections and deaths reached record numbers. The official numbers of dead may never be known, as many died at home and were not recorded.

Testing and Treatment

When COVID-19 began spreading across North America and Europe in March 2020, each country seemed to have a different strategy when it came to testing citizens for the virus. Because it was such a new virus, governments did not have the supplies they needed to test everyone.

As some countries secured the supplies needed for mass testing, every person with any symptom of COVID-19 was encouraged to get tested. Even after vaccines were developed, some countries continued to prioritize testing. During the third wave, the United Kingdom (UK) rolled out at-home testing kits. Thay was a way for them to monitor the virus and continue to track it, even though many UK citizens had been vaccinated.

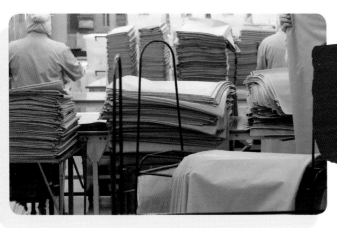

Gloves, masks, and other PPE were often rationed, or limited, during the first wave of the COVID-19 pandemic.

South Korea's Testing Strategy

South Korea adopted a different testing strategy from the very beginning. Its government focused its resources on maximizing testing capacity and offering free tests to every person. The South Korean government learned valuable lessons from previous disease outbreaks such as MERS. It applied them to COVID-19 testing and contact tracing. Starting in January 2020, South Korean officials urged local **biotech** companies to start producing testing kits. Within a month, the country was testing more than 10,000 people every day.

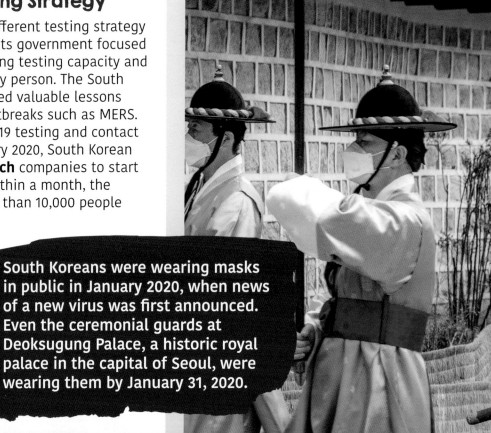

South Koreans were wearing masks in public in January 2020, when news of a new virus was first announced. Even the ceremonial guards at Deoksugung Palace, a historic royal palace in the capital of Seoul, were wearing them by January 31, 2020.

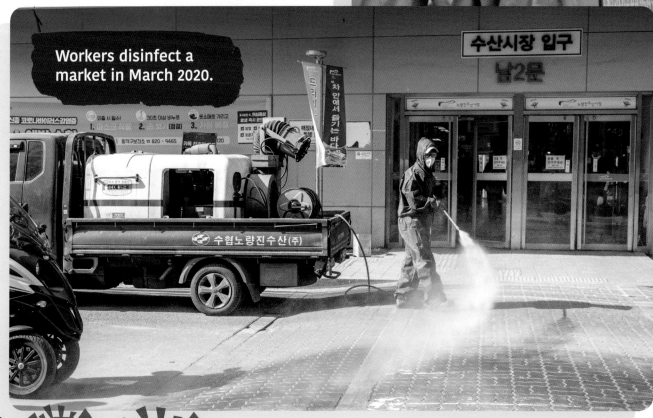

Workers disinfect a market in March 2020.

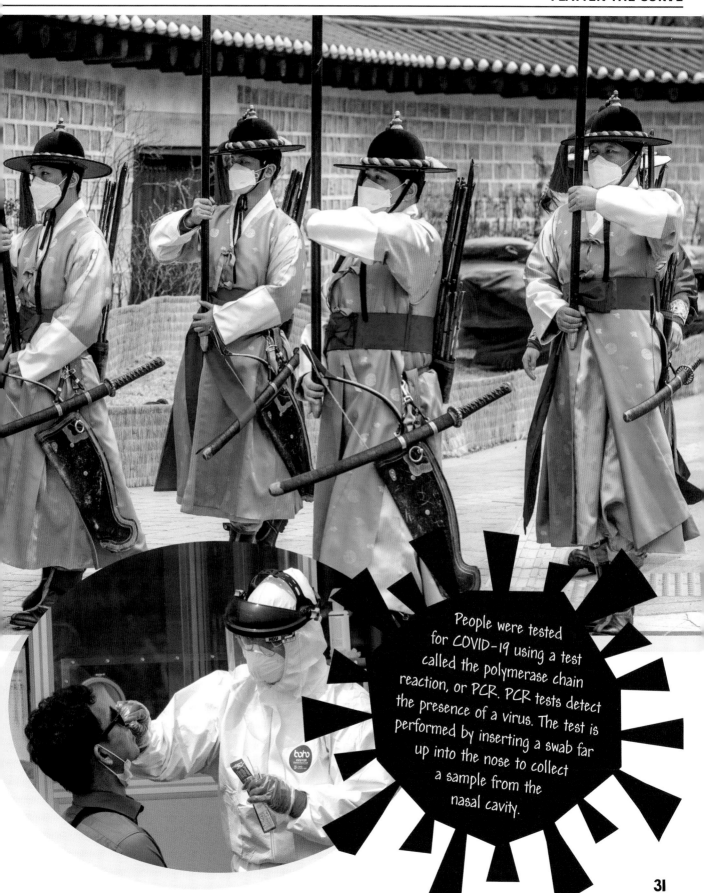

People were tested for COVID-19 using a test called the polymerase chain reaction, or PCR. PCR tests detect the presence of a virus. The test is performed by inserting a swab far up into the nose to collect a sample from the nasal cavity.

New Treatments

Treating patients with a previously unknown disease is tough. At the beginning, health care workers did everything they could just to keep their COVID-19 patients alive. Over time, as medical professionals learned more about COVID-19, they began to discover better treatment options. A ventilator is a machine that helps people breathe when they cannot do so on their own. As COVID-19 spread around the world, ventilators were in short supply. Governments raced to secure them. Doctors around the world sounded alarm bells that they did not have enough of these lifesaving machines.

In the United States, manufacturing, securing, and distributing ventilators became a major effort. By the second and third waves, many countries had ventilators they were not using. Some gave or loaned them to other areas that were in need.

It takes a long time to vaccinate billions of people. There are so many things to consider, such as how to deliver the vaccines, how to give them out to the public, and how to make sure everyone who wants one can have one.

A nurse checks a patient's ventilator. COVID-19 can cause a condition called acute respiratory distress syndrome (ARDS). ARDS reduces the lungs' ability to provide organs with oxygen.

Vaccine Research

From the start of the pandemic, one goal that never changed was finding a vaccine that would offer protection from the virus or lessen its impact. While medical research is usually kept confidential, the research for a COVID-19 vaccine was different. This is because creating a vaccine was a common goal for all governments and drug companies. Using high-tech scientific knowledge and technology, Chinese scientists determined SARS-CoV-2's **genetic structure** very early in the pandemic. This information was shared with scientists all over the world—allowing them to create a number of different vaccines in record time. On November 9, 2020, media outlets announced three vaccines. Those and later vaccines would help reduce the virus's spread and lessen its effects.

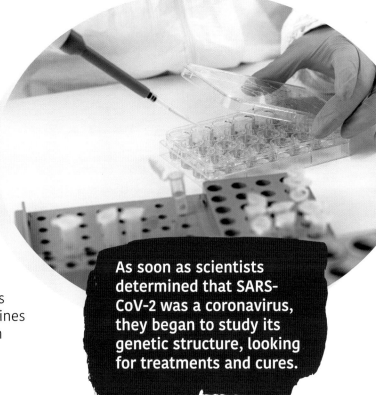

As soon as scientists determined that SARS-CoV-2 was a coronavirus, they began to study its genetic structure, looking for treatments and cures.

PANDEMIC HERO

Dr. Lorna Breen

Dr. Lorna Breen was an emergency room physician at the Columbia University Irving Medical Center and New York-Presbyterian Hospital. In the first months of the pandemic, Breen worked 18-hour days treating COVID-19 patients. She told her family that there were "so many sick people everywhere." Some were dying in the waiting room before they even got into a hospital room. Dr. Breen slept in hospital hallways, rarely going home. Eventually, Dr. Breen contracted the illness herself. She fought COVID-19 and survived, but when she tried to come back to work to support her colleagues, she just didn't have the strength to last a full shift. Dr. Breen took her own life on April 26, 2020. While she did not die directly from COVID-19, her family believes that the effects of the virus combined with the situation at work made her another victim of the pandemic.

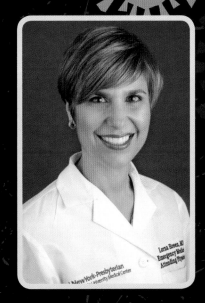

Dr. Breen worked in New York during the deadly first wave of COVID-19. She and thousands of other medical workers risked their lives, and suffered exhaustion and depression after seeing so many patients they cared for die.

Strategies Moving Forward

The COVID-19 pandemic is not the first pandemic the world has seen. Unfortunately, it will also not be the last. Looking at pandemics from the past can help us understand the way that governments around the world have responded to COVID-19.

Epidemiologists are the scientists who study diseases and their spread. For decades, they have been saying that the world was "due" for another major pandemic. The WHO's website is packed with documents that talk about the risk of a new pandemic and how the world should be preparing. In 2015, Bill Gates, the founder of computer technology company Microsoft and head of the **Bill & Melinda Gates Foundation**, gave a **TED Talk** on pandemics. He said the next major threat to the global population wasn't war, like it was when he was young. Instead, he predicted that the next big threat would be a new illness that was contagious and dangerous. He said it would be one that we didn't know anything about.

Scientists who study infectious diseases know that new **pathogens** emerge every year—especially ones like SARS-CoV-2 that evolve from animals to humans. They are always asking "what's next?"

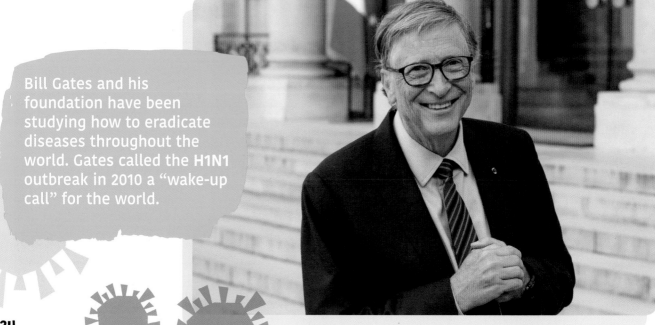

Bill Gates and his foundation have been studying how to eradicate diseases throughout the world. Gates called the **H1N1** outbreak in 2010 a "wake-up call" for the world.

Viruses Threaten All

Gates spoke a lot about the **Ebola** virus outbreaks in 2014 and 2015. He said the problem was that there was no system at all in place to fight this disease and contain its spread. The disease, its impacts, and how it spread had been studied during previous outbreaks. Scientists had learned how to diagnose it, and what treatments to use. For years, many had worked on an Ebola vaccine and had even produced one for human testing. However, there was no pharmaceutical company interested in developing the vaccine because it cost too much. Before it reached American shores in 2014, there was little interest in the virus. Ebola was considered a disease of tropical countries, and it had killed just 1,300 people in 30 years.

Back in 2015, Gates told the world that "the failure to prepare could allow the next epidemic to be dramatically more devastating than Ebola."

The WHO made its disease monitoring better since the Ebola outbreaks. Rapid response has improved in many countries, as well. But COVID-19 proved few were ready for a virus that could be spread rapidly by people who showed no symptoms.

The Bill & Melinda Gates Foundation is a co-founder of the Coalition for Epidemic Preparedness Innovations (CEPI). This organization helps fund vaccine creation for new viruses. CEPI gave millions for SARS-CoV-2 vaccine research in 2020—21. It sees new coronaviruses as serious threats to public health. Some see CEPI's work as important, but believe it puts too much power in the hands of drug companies that control vaccine supplies. This could lead to more **unequal distribution** of vaccines. Poorer countries would suffer because the emphasis would be on making money, rather than sharing vaccine formulas and saving lives.

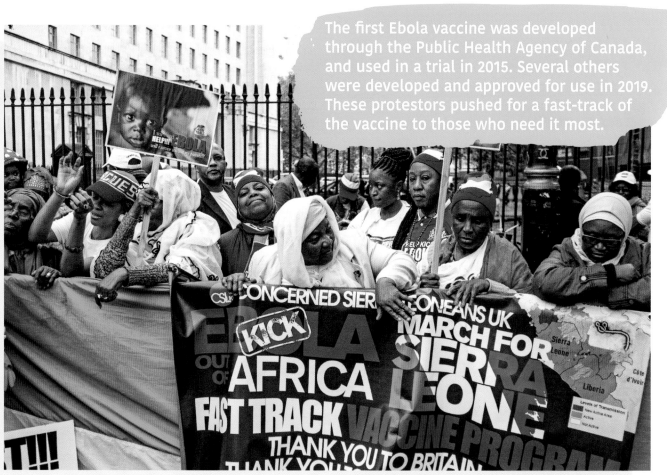

The first Ebola vaccine was developed through the Public Health Agency of Canada, and used in a trial in 2015. Several others were developed and approved for use in 2019. These protestors pushed for a fast-track of the vaccine to those who need it most.

Comparing Past Pandemics

Governments around the world had fought pandemics before. Many pandemics of the past were more deadly than COVID-19 because there were no vaccines or life-saving treatments. But none hit every corner of the world quite like COVID-19.

The 1918-19 Flu

The 1918–1919 pandemic is also known as the Spanish Flu because it was first widely reported in Spain. Scientists say the flu did not begin there. It was caused by a virus that researchers believe originated from a bird. The Spanish flu killed 50 million people around the world, and 675,000 of those in the United States alone. This flu spread in similar ways to COVID-19, but hit the young even more than the elderly. In 1918, medicine was not as advanced as it is now. There were few effective drugs and no life-saving ventilators. The Spanish flu also spread widely when soldiers returned home from **World War I**.

Just like today, governments tried to limit the spread of the Spanish flu. They recommended that people isolate, quarantine, limit public gatherings, and wear masks.

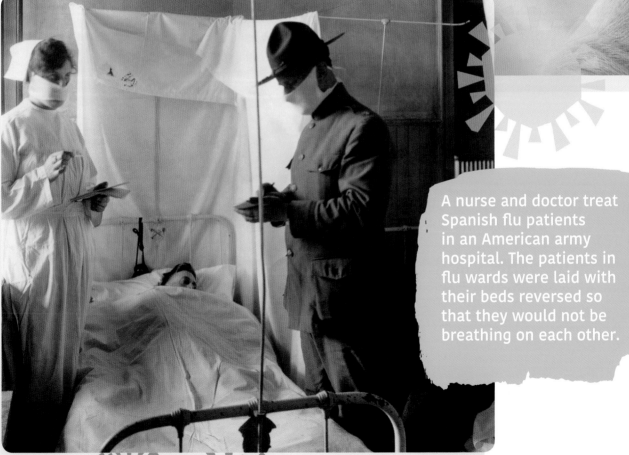

A nurse and doctor treat Spanish flu patients in an American army hospital. The patients in flu wards were laid with their beds reversed so that they would not be breathing on each other.

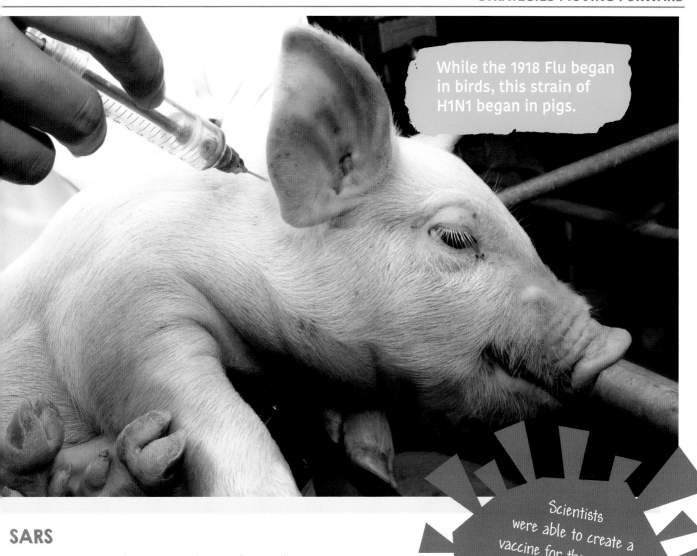

While the 1918 Flu began in birds, this strain of H1N1 began in pigs.

Scientists were able to create a vaccine for the swine flu quite quickly. On August 10, 2020, the WHO declared an end to the 2009 H1N1 pandemic.

SARS

Severe acute respiratory syndrome, better known as SARS, is a virus caused by a coronavirus called SARS-CoV. It was first reported in China in November 2002. It spread to 29 countries before the outbreak was contained. SARS was far more deadly than COVID-19, but it didn't spread as easily. People infected with SARS were so sick most could not travel. That often kept them away from others, and prevented them from spreading the disease. SARS could only be spread when a person showed symptoms of the disease.

The Swine Flu

In 2009, another pandemic was caused by a new strain of the H1N1 virus. It began in Mexico, but was then discovered and identified in the United States. It quickly spread across the country and to many countries around the world. While it was a new strain of H1N1, people who had been exposed to previous H1N1 viruses seemed to have some sort of immunity. Because of that, the disease infected more young people than old. The CDC estimated that between April 2009 and April 2010, there were 60.8 million cases of H1N1 and 12,469 deaths in the United States. There were up to 575,400 deaths worldwide.

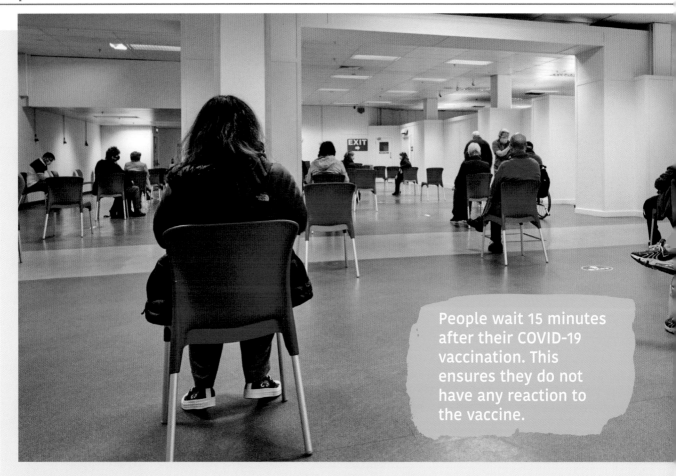

People wait 15 minutes after their COVID-19 vaccination. This ensures they do not have any reaction to the vaccine.

Herd Immunity

Herd immunity was another term mentioned almost daily during the COVID-19 pandemic. Herd immunity occurs when most of a population is immune to an infectious disease. But what does that mean? Being immune to a disease means that your body has a layer of protection inside that prevents you from becoming infected. When most of a population has immunity to a disease, the disease runs out of hosts. Eventually, without hosts, it dies. When COVID-19 spread across the world, it was a new illness, so no one had immunity to it. To stop the spread, herd immunity would be required.

For example, when 80 percent of a group of people is immune to a virus, that means four out of every five people who are exposed to the virus won't get sick. They also won't spread the virus to others. That keeps the spread under control. Every virus is different, but typically 50 to 90 percent of a population needs to be immune to the virus to achieve herd immunity.

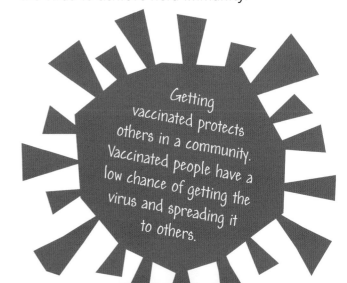

Getting vaccinated protects others in a community. Vaccinated people have a low chance of getting the virus and spreading it to others.

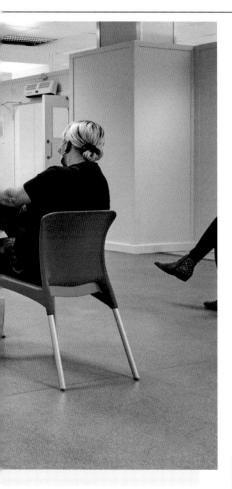

How to Get There

There are different ways of achieving herd immunity in a population. The first, and most dangerous, is to simply let a virus run its course and infect a lot of people. With most viruses, once a person becomes infected and recovers, their body creates **antibodies**. These protect them from catching the disease again, making them immune. The problem with this method of achieving herd immunity is that a lot of people may die, and more people need care from hospitals.

Vaccinations

The second method of achieving herd immunity is by vaccinating a population. Vaccinations have helped limit the spread of many formerly common diseases such as measles and rubella. Some diseases, such as smallpox, have been eradicated, or destroyed, by vaccinations. Most people alive today receive vaccinations at a young age. Those vaccinations protect the population from a variety of diseases that once killed people or made them very sick. COVID-19 vaccines were quickly developed so that herd immunity could be achieved.

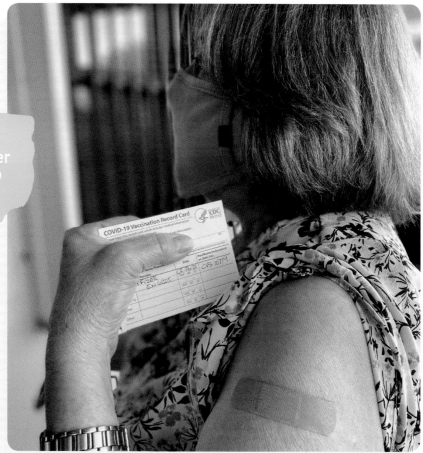

A woman shows her vaccination card after getting her COVID-19 vaccination.

Illness and Immunity

Herd immunity is the best way to overcome an infectious disease, but it's certainly not perfect. First, any time a person develops immunity to a disease, there are questions around how long the immunity lasts. COVID-19 is a new disease that hit the world so quickly and with great force. It was more difficult to combat because there was so little known about it. Based on what scientists knew about other diseases, they assumed that once a person recovered from COVID-19 they were immune for some time. However, COVID-19 was different. Some people contracted it more than once.

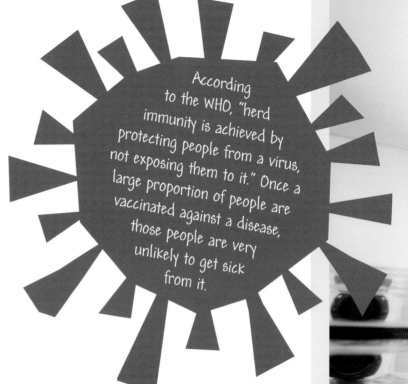

According to the WHO, "herd immunity is achieved by protecting people from a virus, not exposing them to it." Once a large proportion of people are vaccinated against a disease, those people are very unlikely to get sick from it.

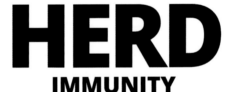

HERD
IMMUNITY
COVID-19

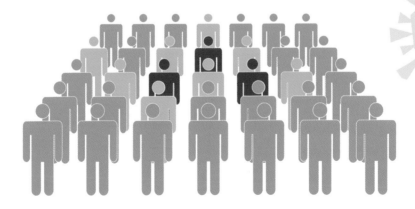

INFECTIOUS AGENT PASSES FREELY
FROM CONTAGIOUS TO SUSCEPTIBLE

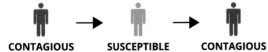

CONTAGIOUS   SUSCEPTIBLE   CONTAGIOUS

CONTAGION CANNOT FREELY PASS
VIA IMMUNISED TO SUSCEPTIBLE

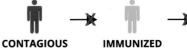

CONTAGIOUS   IMMUNIZED   SUSCEPTIBLE

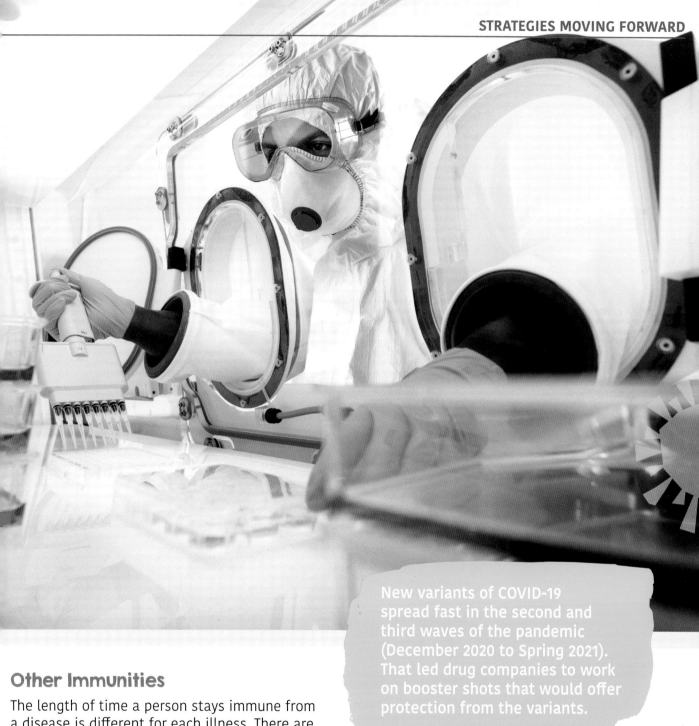

New variants of COVID-19 spread fast in the second and third waves of the pandemic (December 2020 to Spring 2021). That led drug companies to work on booster shots that would offer protection from the variants.

Other Immunities

The length of time a person stays immune from a disease is different for each illness. There are four common coronaviruses. They cause 15 to 30 percent of common colds. With these viruses, a person is immune for one to two years after they recover. That means for a year or two, that person will not catch the same virus again. If enough people also become immune to a virus at the same time, herd immunity is achieved and the virus would become much less common around the world.

One of the things that scared the world most about COVID-19 was that nobody knew how to achieve immunity. Then, once immunity was achieved, no one knew how long it would last. That's why it became clear that the only way to beat this virus was to develop a vaccine.

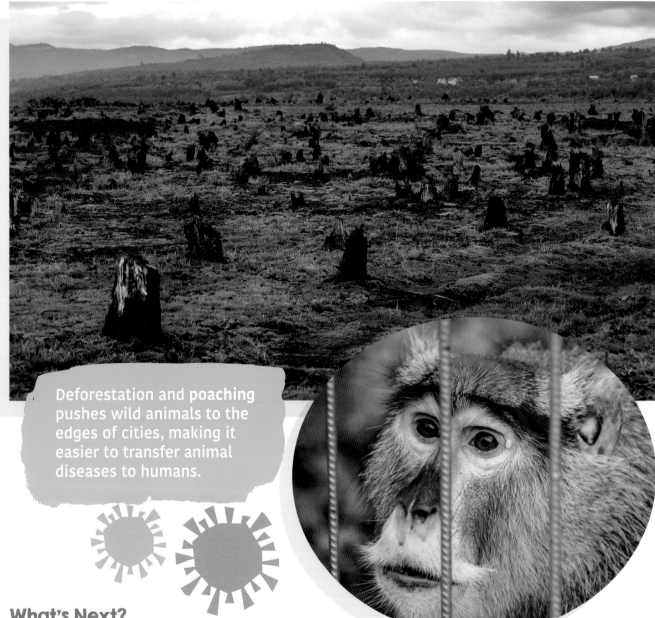

Deforestation and **poaching** pushes wild animals to the edges of cities, making it easier to transfer animal diseases to humans.

What's Next?

Scientists predict that there will be more pandemics in the future. They are already laying out plans to prevent them. That will not be easy. The world population is growing by 1.1 percent per year. That many not seem like a lot, but this small percentage means that every year, the population of the world grows by 83 million people. More people means less space, which leads to overcrowded cities. The United Nations predicts that by 2050, two out of three people in the world will be living in cities. With more and more people living in smaller spaces, infectious diseases are easier to spread.

Zoonotic Diseases

Many of the world's pandemics began from zoonotic viruses. Those viruses came from animals and eventually changed in a way that let them infect humans. Rapid deforestation happening around the world is destroying animal habitats and pushing animals closer together. Increases in factory farming techniques that keep many animals in small, cramped spaces also provide a perfect environment for viruses to spread between animals.

International Travel

The world is very reliant on international travel. Thay means keeping any illness or disease from spreading between countries is nearly impossible. When COVID-19 is under control and the world settles into a new form of normal, more people will once again begin crossing borders for work or tourism. That again will increase the chances of a virus spreading.

Better Science

The positive thing is that there is better science, better technology, and better coordination in the world today than ever before. International communication can play a large role in preventing a pandemic like COVID-19 from happening again. Governments must communicate with one another and warn the rest of the world of new viruses infecting their populations. To prevent the next pandemic from having the same devastating impacts as COVID-19, governments and their people must take these warnings seriously. People need to learn what worked and what didn't work to slow the spread of the disease.

A COVID-19 safety precautions sign on a trail in California reminds people to be respectful of others trying to social distance.

Travelers wait for flights in airports in seats that have green checkmarks for approved distancing.

43

Bibliography

Introduction

Baraniuk, Chris. "What the Diamond Princess taought the world about COVID-19." BMJ, April 27, 2020.
https://www.bmj.com/content/369/bmj.m1632

Chapter 1

"Countries." The World Health Organization.
https://www.who.int/countries

Kassam, Ashifa. "113-year-old coronavirus survivor: 'The elderly are the forgotten ones of society.'" The Guardian, May 16, 2020.
https://www.theguardian.com/world/2020/may/16/worlds-oldest-coronavirus-survivor-the-elderly-are-the-forgotten-ones-of-society

"Mission, Role and Pledge." Centers for Disease Control and Prevention, May 13, 2019.
https://www.cdc.gov/about/organization/mission.htm

"Older Adults." Centers for Disease Control and Prevention, June 9, 2021.
https://www.cdc.gov/coronavirus/2019-ncov/need-extra-precautions/older-adults.html

Chapter 2

"Common Colds: Protect Yourself and Others." Centers for Disease Control and Prevention, October 7, 2020.
https://www.cdc.gov/features/rhinoviruses/index.html

Draulans, Dirk. 'Finally, a virus got me.' Scientist who fought Ebola and HIV reflects on facing death from COVID-19." Science, May 8, 2020.
https://bit.ly/3tJQww1

Ducharme, Jamie. "World Health Organization Declares COVID-19 a 'Pandemic.' Here's What That Means." Time Magazine, March 11, 2020.
https://www.sciencemag.org/news/2020/05/finally-virus-got-me-scientist-who-fought-ebola-and-hiv-reflects-facing-death-covid-19

Mesel-Lemoine, M., et al. "A Human Coronavirus Responsible for the Common Cold Massively Kills Dendritic Cells but Not Monocytes." Jour. of Virology, July 2012.
https://www.ncbi.nlm.nih.gov/pmc/articles/PMC3416289/

"SARS Basics Fact Sheet." Centers for Disease Control and Prevention, December 6, 2017.
https://www.cdc.gov/sars/about/fs-sars.html

Chapter 3

Bjorklund, K., and A. Ewing. "The Swedish COVID-19 Response Is a Disaster. It Shouldn't Be a Model for the Rest of the World." Time Magazine, Oct. 14, 2020.
https://bit.ly/3p7jpP6

Boserup, Brad, et al. "Alarming trends in US domestic violence during the COVID-19 pandemic." American Journal of Emergency Medicine, Apr. 28, 2020.
https://www.ncbi.nlm.nih.gov/pmc/articles/PMC7195322/

"COVID Data Tracker." Centers for Disease Control and Prevention.
https://covid.cdc.gov/covid-data-tracker/#datatracker-home

Ellis, S. "Tsai Ing-wen, Taiwan's Covid Crusher. Businessweek, Dec. 3, 2020.
https://www.bloomberg.com/news/articles/2020-12-03/tsai-ing-wen-taiwan-s-covid-crusher-bloomberg-50-2020

Hudson, Hayley. "Recent Statistics Show Opioid Addiction And COVID-19 Dangers. Addiction Center, August 13, 2020.
https://www.addictioncenter.com/community/recent-statistics-show-opioid-addiction-covid-19-dangers/

Jones, Sam, and Ashifa Kassam. "Spain defends response to coronavirus as global cases exceed 500,000." The Guardian, March 26, 2020.
https://www.theguardian.com/world/2020/mar/26/spanish-coronavirus-deaths-slow-as-world-nears-500000-cases

"Mortality Analyses." Johns Hopkins University of Medicine, June 11, 2021.
https://coronavirus.jhu.edu/data/mortality

Pingyuan Lu, E. "Taiwan, Sweden showing the world." Taipei Times, May 21, 2020.
https://www.taipeitimes.com/News/editorials/archives/2020/05/21/2003736770

Sandford, Alasdair. "Coronavirus: Half of humanity now on lockdown as 90 countries call for confinement." Euronews, April 3, 2020.
https://www.euronews.com/2020/04/02/coronavirus-in-europe-spain-s-death-toll-hits-10-000-after-record-950-new-deaths-in-24-hou

Taub, Amanda. "A New Covid-19 Crisis: Domestic Abuse Rises Worldwide." The New York Times, April 6, 2020.
https://www.nytimes.com/2020/04/06/world/coronavirus-domestic-violence.html

"United States Unemployment Rate." Trading Economics.
https://tradingeconomics.com/united-states/unemployment-rate

Vogel, Gretchen. "It's been so, so surreal.' Critics of Sweden's lax pandemic policies face fierce backlash." Science, Oct. 6, 2020.
https://www.sciencemag.org/news/2020/10/it-s-been-so-so-surreal-critics-sweden-s-lax-pandemic-policies-face-fierce-backlash

Chapter 4

"Gillespie, Claire. "Proning Is a Promising Treatment for Coronavirus—Here's How It Works." Health, April 21, 2020.
https://www.health.com/condition/infectious-diseases/coronavirus/proning-treatment-coronavirus

Horowitz, Jason. "Italy's Health Care System Groans Under Coronavirus – a Warning to the World." The New York Times, March 12, 2020.
https://www.nytimes.com/2020/03/12/world/europe/12italy-coronavirus-health-care.html

Ornstein, Charles. "How America's Hospitals Survived the First Wave of the Coronavirus." ProPublica, June 15, 2020.
https://www.propublica.org/article/how-americas-hospitals-survived-the-first-wave-of-the-coronavirus

Wang, Jessica, et al. "How China Built Two Coronavirus Hospitals in Just Over a Week." The Wall Street Journal, February 6, 2020.
https://www.wsj.com/articles/how-china-can-build-a-coronavirus-hospital-in-10-days-11580397751

Watkins, Ali, et al. "Top E.R. Doctor Who Treated Virus Patients Dies by Suicide." The New York Times, April 27, 2020.
https://www.nytimes.com/2020/04/27/nyregion/new-york-city-doctor-suicide-coronavirus.html

Zastrow, Mark. "How South Korea prevented a coronavirus disaster—and why the battle isn't over." National Geographic, May 12, 2020.
https://www.nationalgeographic.com/science/article/how-south-korea-prevented-coronavirus-disaster-why-battle-is-not-over

Chapter 5

"1918 Pandemic (H1N1 Virus)." Centers for Disease Control and Prevention, March 20, 2019.
https://www.cdc.gov/flu/pandemic-resources/1918-pandemic-h1n1.html

"2009 H1N1 Pandemic (H1N1pdm09 virus)." Centers for Disease Control and Prevention, June 11, 2019.
https://www.cdc.gov/flu/pandemic-resources/1918-pandemic-h1n1.html

"A Chronicle on the SARS Epidemic." Chinese Law and Government, December 7, 2014.
https://www.tandfonline.com/doi/abs/10.2753/CLG0009-4609360412?journalCode=mclg20

"Coronavirus disease (COVID-19): Herd immunity, lockdowns and COVID-19." The World Health Organization, December 31, 2020.
https://www.who.int/news-room/q-a-detail/herd-immunity-lockdowns-and-covid-19

Gates, Bill. "The next outbreak? We're not ready." TED Talks.
https://bit.ly/377QcgL

Lee, Harold K.K., et al. "Asymptomatic Severe Acute Respiratory Syndrome–associated Coronavirus Infection." Emerging Infectious Diseases, November 2003.https://www.ted.com/talks/bill_gates_the_next_outbreak_we_re_not_ready/transcript?language=en

Twohey, M., and N. Kulish. "Bill Gates, the Virus and the Quest to Vaccinate the World." The New York Times, May 8, 2021.
https://www.nytimes.com/2020/11/23/world/bill-gates-vaccine-coronavirus.html

Timeline

December 10, 2019 One of the first suspected coronavirus patients falls ill in China.

December 30, 2019 Wuhan doctor Li Wenliang shares information about the new virus online.

December 31, 2019 Chinese authorities alert WHO of an outbreak of pneumonia cases in Wuhan, China.

January 9, 2020 WHO announces Chinese outbreak is caused by novel coronavirus.

January 21, 2020 CDC confirms the first coronavirus case in the United States.

January 23, 2020 Wuhan, China is put into lockdown.

January 24, 2020 China extends its lockdown to include 36 million people.

March 11, 2020 WHO declares COVID-19 a pandemic and calls for global response to contain it.

April 4, 2020 More than 1 million cases of COVID-19 are confirmed worldwide.

September 4, 2020 Early phase trial results of Russia's Sputnik V vaccine are announced.

December 14, 2020 Canada administers its first COVID-19 vaccine.

December 23, 2020 The United States reaches 1 million vaccinations, with 150 million fully vaccinated by June 2021.

May 4, 2021 154 million COVID-19 cases are reported worldwide.

June 22, 2021 The WHO says the Delta variant of COVID-19 is becoming dominant.

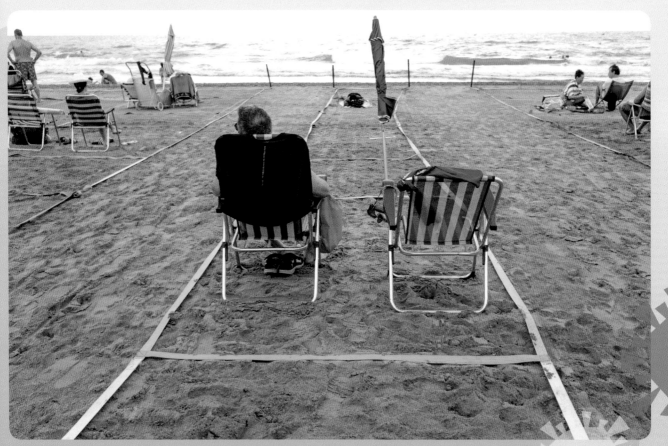

Learning More

Books

Naik, Anant. *Heroes of a Pandemic: Those who stood up against COVID-19*. Indy Pub, 2020.

O'Brien, Cynthia. *The War Against COVID-19*. Crabtree Publishing, 2021.

O'Neal, Claire. *The Influenza Pandemic of 1918*. Mitchell Lane. February, 2020.

Websites

Tips from the Centers for Disease Control and Prevention on strategies teens and young adults can take to manage their stress during COVID-19.
https://www.cdc.gov/coronavirus/2019-ncov/daily-life-coping/stress-coping/young-adults.html

Resources to help young people cope with COVID-19 including videos and audio mediations. Readers can see how the virus and disease spread and what actions were taken.
https://www.aboutkidshealth.ca/COVID-19

A kid-friendly guide to the science of coronaviruses and COVID-19, including understanding viruses and cells.
https://www.livescience.com/coronavirus-kids-guide.html

Glossary

airborne Carried through the air

antibodies Proteins in the blood gained through an exposure to an illness that protect from becoming infected with the illness again

Bill & Melinda Gates Foundation The largest private charitable foundation in the world, dedicated to funding health care and reducing poverty

biotech Short for biotechnology, the field of biology in which products such as medicines and vaccines are developed

cells The smallest unit of an organism; all living beings are made out of cells

chronic Continuing or happening again and again for a long time

contained Kept under control

contact tracing The process of identifying those who have come in contact with a person diagnosed with an infectious disease

contagious Likely to spread between people

Glossary

curfews Orders requiring people to be home and off the streets at a certain time

deforestation The practice of clearing large areas of trees

Ebola A deadly disease that causes bleeding

evolved Developed or changed into something different

exponential spread Very rapid spread over time

first wave The first mass groups to contract the virus

genetic structure The pattern or makeup that contains information about a living thing

global warming The gradual warming of Earth's temperature caused by human activity

HINI A type of flu virus known as swine flu

hosts Plants, animals, or people on which another organism lives

infectious Likely to spread

lockdowns Rules put in place by the government to limit people's activities to reduce the spread of disease

microscopic Seen only with a microscope

non-essential Not absolutely necessary

opioid A type of very addictive drug

pandemic A disease outbreak spread over a large area such as a country, a continent, or the world

pathogens Viruses, bacteria, and other tiny organisms that cause disease

poaching Illegal hunting of wild animals

protocols A system of rules and procedures that are followed so that things run smoothly

public health Health services that protect a community or a country

quarantine Imposed isolation when a person may have been exposed to, or has, a disease

reproduce Have offspring

respiratory Relating to the lungs and breathing

respiratory droplets Small, liquid droplets of saliva or mucous produced by breathing, speaking, or singing

social distancing Maintaining distance between people to prevent the spread of an illness

state of emergency A situation of urgent need, such as a disaster, that is declared by the government to keep people safe

symptoms A physical or mental change or feeling of illness caused by being infected with a disease

TED Talks An American media organization that posts talks on many subjects online for free distribution

unequal distribution When something is given out to people in an uneven or unfair way

unhoused Having no shelter or place to live

variants Changes in a virus that have occured over time when the virus replicates itself

visas Official documents or passport stamps that allow people to enter, stay in, or leave a country

World Health Organization (WHO) A United Nations agency that looks after public health issues all over the world

World War I A war between the world's great powers and their allies (1914–1918) fought mainly in Europe and the Middle East

Index

About the Author

Samantha Kohn is a professional writer who moved to working from home during the COVID-19 pandemic. She built a gym in her basement and spent most of her spare time going on marathon-length walks. She also had a wedding during the pandemic, marrying an emergency room nurse working on the frontlines of the pandemic.